CHOOSING THE SEX OF YOUR BABY, GOD'S METHOD

By

Rev'd Vincent Uzomah Obibuaku

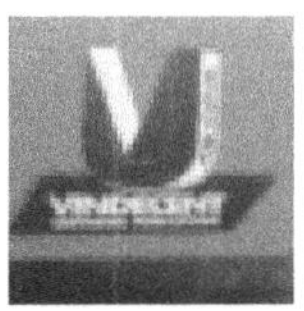

VINDECENT UNIVERSAL PUBLICATION

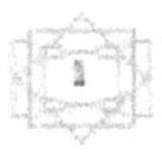

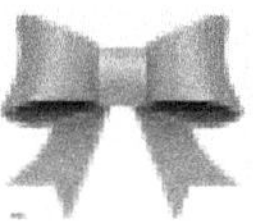

DEDICATION

This book is dedicated to God Almighty, without whom I would not have imagined that a book of this kind will be written by me; and also to my wife and Children. I own you a debt of love and faithfulness.

To God be the glory.

TABLE OF CONTENT

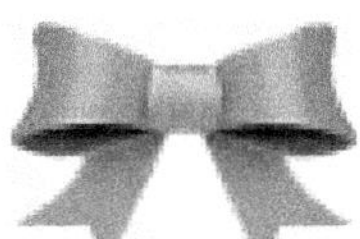

INTRODUCTION

In a world where scientific advancements have opened the door to various methods of selecting the `sex of a baby, "Divine Decisions" takes a unique perspective. This is to enable us see from the spiritual and religious dimensions of this crucial decision. Delving into the intersection of faith and family planning. We shall be provided with a thoughtful and insightful guide to help us, as we seek to understand and embrace "God's Method" for choosing the sex of our baby.

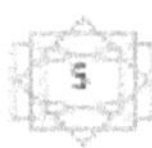

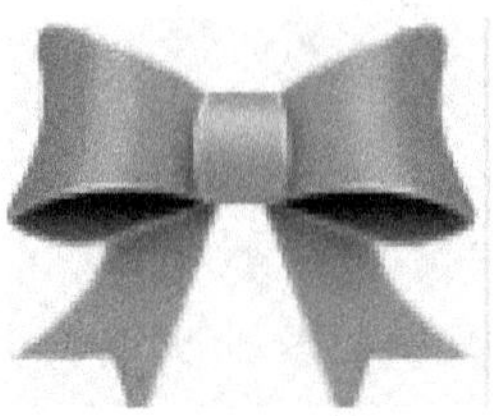

PREFACE

As the pursuit of parenthood evolves, so too does the profound desire to align these decisions with one's faith, seeking divine guidance in the sacred journey of bringing forth life.

Choosing the Sex of Your Baby, God's Method, embarks on a thoughtful exploration, through experience to bring couples who are cut in this web, into a realm where the spiritual tapestry of existence weaves seamlessly with the intricate fabric of family planning. In the midst of the struggles faced by both the devout believers and those that are not, in finding God's will and intervention in regard to having a male or female child. this book endeavours to offer a compass as you navigate through the delicate terrain between fertility issues and prayers.

Reverend Vincent U. Obibuaku.

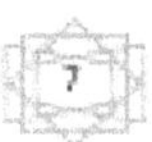

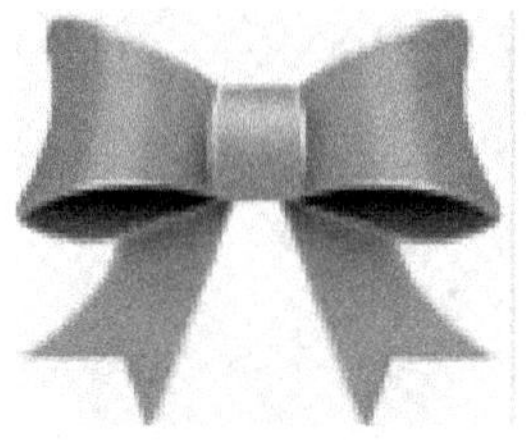

CHAPTER ONE

GOD'S PLAN FOR THE HOME

The home is a complete and beautiful place that God made. God did put all things needed to bring in completeness, in other to make the home a joyous and happy place, with nothing missing. It was not until Satan entered the home of the first man and woman "Adam and Eve", and altered this plan of God on marriage.

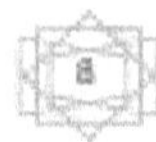

It is not that Satan is supreme over God in this case. No, God is. But the issue is, Satan always work with man's "lack of knowledge" to overcome him in areas where he lacks them. 'Knowledge they say is power' and God has said in his word that "My people' are destroyed for lack of knowledge" (Hosea 4:6).

If we fail to apply knowledge (reasoning) where it is needed, God himself, except when He want to intervene. Will leave us with our choice, and we face the consequences. God has given man knowledge, sense of reasoning, to act like Him.

"I said, ye are gods, and all of you sons of the Most High. Ps 82:6, ASV.

When God made the woman, He brought her to the man. It was him (man) himself that confirmed it, when he said, "This is now the bone of my bones and flesh of my flesh; she shall be called woman, 'because' she was taken out of man" Genesis 2:23. (this statement was made out of reasoning).

"If you seek [Wisdom] as for silver and search for skillful and godly Wisdom as for hidden

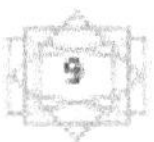

treasures, Then, you will understand the reverent and worshipful fear of the Lord and find the knowledge of [our omniscient] God. For the Lord gives skillful and godly Wisdom; from His mouth come knowledge and understanding. He hides away sound and godly Wisdom and stores it for the righteous (those who are upright and in right standing with Him); He is a shield to those who walk uprightly and in integrity" Proverb. 2:4-7 AMP.

The reverent and worshipful fear of the Lord is the beginning and the principal and choice part of knowledge [it's starting point and its essence]; but fools despise skillful and godly Wisdom, instruction, and discipline." AMP Proverb 1:7

The reverent fear and worship of the Lord is the beginning of Wisdom and skill [the preceding and the first essential, the prerequisite and the alphabet]; a good understanding, wisdom, and meaning have all those who do [the will of the Lord]. Their praise of Him endures forever "Psalm 111:10 AMP.

If anyone despise knowledge, he or she is at his or her own risk, knowledge is the primary thing every child of God should operate in, knowledge of God first equates the knowledge of the things he created for his pleasures. It's the starting point and it's essential, it's the preceding and the first essential, the prerequisite and the alphabet.

Since this plan of God for the home was altered, the home continued to face diverse challenges. Many homes have been on constant attack, some missing out most of the things needed to bring completeness in it.

Several things help to bring completeness to the home. This is because, 'The gift of God makes rich and adds no sorrow,' and we must continue to thank God in whatever situation we find ourselves and in whatever He has given to us. We must as a matter of truth be joyful always, if we must get the attention of God to respond to our needs.

The blessing of the Lord — it makes [truly] rich, and He adds no sorrow with it [neither does toiling increase it]. Proverbs 10:22 AMP. "Be joyful always; pray continually; give

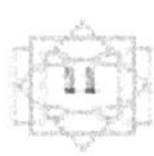

thanks in all circumstances, for this is God's will for you in Christ Jesus." 1 Thessalonians 5:16-18.

The most and the first thing that makes the home complete is happiness. Every couples returning home expects to be made happy on arrival; and the things that ensure this happiness are found in the home not outside. It's found within the hearts and mind of couples. It's a fulfilled home, a home where everything needed to ensure happiness is found. The chief among all is children, the fruit of marriage. "Children are a heritage from the Lord, the fruit of the womb is a reward" Psalm 127:3

Companionship is the primary purpose of breaking loneliness in both the man and woman as it were from creation. There are other things that make up the home or family unit and children are at the center. When children start arriving in the home, their arrival increase the blissfulness and joy of both the couples and the extended family members; sense of fulfillment, adequacy, realness and safety is brought in and instilled. This is not to say that couples who is still waiting on God for children are outside of God's will, plan or enemies with Him. No, No, far be it from me to suggest so. God said in Jeremiah 29:11 **"For I know the thoughts that I think toward you, saith the LORD, thoughts of peace, and not of evil, to give you an expected end. {expected...: Heb. end and expectation}"** (KJV). For couples yet to have their own babies, the Lord knows the best plans He has for them which no man can stop, they are to patiently wait on Him and

In typical African societies according to Michael Oladele, "Lack of children from couples creates tension and worries in homes. Even where there are children, the absence of at least a male child worsens an already tense situation. The female spouse especially feels so insecure in the marriage that the joy and happiness in the home often disappears."

From the Biblical point of view and as believers this shouldn't be the case. God is the giver of children and couples should not blame themselves, if children have not arrived or a situation where couples have only female or male children. They should trust God for His will in their life, because if God's will be not in your plan, He leaves you in the midst thereof to accomplish it.

Jesus said in Matthew 26:39. "O my Father, if it is possible, lets, this cup pass from me; nevertheless not as I will, but as you will.

This piece of writing is intended to bridge the gap created by lack of knowledge of God's will, as it regards sex of baby's selection for couples that are ready to have children.

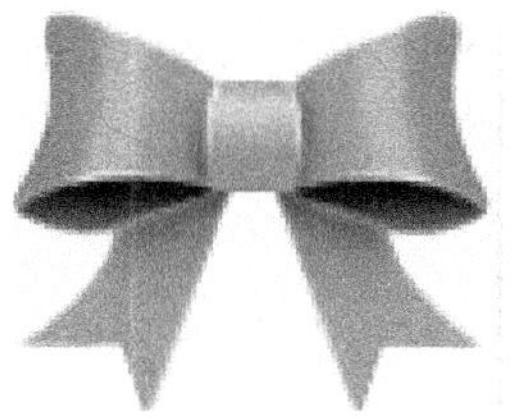

CHAPTER TWO

CHOOSING THE SEX OF A BABY

Many homes today, especially Christian homes struggles with the issues regarding sex of babies, some couples are simply keeping quiet about it, but are dying in silence with no one to break the silence.

God helped me and my wife after our first three children, both of them girls, we had no problems with that, neither did it give us sleepless night, we were happily married, the sex of our children didn't border us, in fact we were grateful to God who gave us three beautiful children.

It was not until sometime age, someone gave my wife a book written by Dr. Shettles, "Choosing the sex of your baby" this book was in our house for almost four years without both of us looking at the content. Not that we cannot read, but the interest in reading a book to choose baby sex, for me, was not a worthwhile thing to do. Because as a devout believer, it is backsliding to think that man has a part to play in sex of baby's selection. it was sinful, even to consider it.

My wife started reading the book, after some time, her interest for the book increased. She started applying what she was learning. She began with the calculation of her menstrual circle and ovulation day and all of that, but could not achieve result. When our third child arrived, it was a girl.

One day my wife asked me to follow her and read the book, she kept insisting that I must

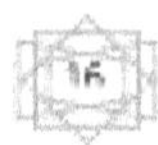

join her in reading it. In other to make her happy, one day I opened the book, after reading the first and second chapters. My attention was drawn to certain principles that is natural, not mechanical nor scientific. Just calculation of timing of when to approach a woman and nothing more, and a deep penetration. I said, ah it could be our fault. We were not following the rules. It is not that God didn't want us to have a male child, we were not simply following his plans and applying the principles aright.

My interest aroused, my gaze into the book intensified, my mind opened, I now realized that it was not what I thought. I went on and on with reading the book, and I came to discover that the major part of the job will have to be done by me in helping my wife to follow the menstrual circle reading and timing, making sure she reaches orgasm and penetrate deep before ejaculation.

I discovered that the man has to learn to wait for the right time before having sex with the woman, especially when expecting to have a baby. That is to say, you time when you can have intercourse with your wife during menstrual circle, because the closer it is to the time of ovulation, the better the chances of having a boy.

The man will have to learn to hold himself and not jump on the wife at any time for sex, he has to help her out here. This understanding is very important between husband and wife.

So God helped us with this knowledge and careful prayers, by the time we had our next child, God gave us a bouncing baby boy.

As I said earlier, we were not worried at all with the gifts of girl children God gave to us, myself and my spouse. No extended family members spoke to me about not having male child, of cause, I expected that from my family. Because they knew me very well and the principles I stood for, so I did not expect any body to approach me about it.

The gender of my children was never a prayer point to me. Rather the things that were of concern to me, where more or less a testimony sort of. I wanted my case to bring glory to God. If it were His will!

Another thing I wanted was, as a marriage counselour, my counselees look up to me. Even though I was not really praying for male child, but because of this, I said oh God do it for me that others may see and by it be comforted.

"God is our merciful Father and the source of all comfort. He comforts us in all our troubles so that we can comfort others. When they are troubled, we will be able to give them the same comfort God has given us." 2 Corinthians 1:3-5. This scripture was my anchor Bible passage in this case.

So as we began to read the book called "choosing the sex of your BABY," No interest, as I said earlier. Choosing the sex of a baby is solely determined by God, man has no part to play.

But the book exposed me to what is called menstrual cycle, ovulation and chromosomes X and Y. I knew little or nothing about counting a woman's cycle. But when I paid attention to the guide lines I discover truly that there are many things God has made; His plans for man, which can only be tapped into by knowledge.

Job said, "I KNOW that my redeemer lives." Job 19: 25. Daniel said, "In the first year of his reign I, Daniel UNDERSTOOD by the books." Daniel 9:2.

One of the things I discovered was the fact that a woman's body is designed in such a way that it works with season or period. The female body is created in a way that it functions seasonally or periodically. There is a time the female body prepares for pregnancy. Mind you, I am not a doctor, but my eye was opened to this fact that I might help you overcome your marital challenges in the area of child bearing. Choosing the sex of your child.

One thing we must know as men is that every day is not the same in a woman's body; we must help our wife to observe these seasons. Everyday maybe for sex but everyday sex may not give you the sex of the baby you need. Husbands are encouraged to assist their wife in ensuring that this record is accurately kept, because it will help you to know when to call for sex and when to abstain.

If the day you want her is outside the date the ovary is ready for the sex of the baby you are expecting, you can easily advice yourself to hold on, of course you know that your wife will not refuse you.

Many men get angry with their wife when they try to refuse them sex, and when the pregnancy comes and it is not the sex they expect; they cast blame on the woman.

For full details about this, get the book; "Choosing the Sex of your Baby" Dr. Shettles Method via:
https://a.co/d/7ZTOkoE
or better still for marriage counseling in regard to this (sex of a baby), or any other marital issues you may have. contact me on my various contact information's.

WhatsApp: 0904541417,
Email: winnetsoul@yahoo.com
https//winnetsoulnetwork.wordpress.com
I WILL GLADLY OFFER MY ADVICE TO HELP YOU.

This information is both for the husbands and his wife, especially the man because he produces the XY chromosome which produces the boy child and while the woman has an XX chromosome which produces the girl child.

It is the man that produces and deposits the sperm cell that determines the sex of the baby and not the woman. So before you jump on her next time, check the season she is in and help create the atmosphere conducive for the preferred Chromosome to fertilize the egg.

The woman must also be able to know the date of her ovulation, adequate knowledge of one's ovulation day will help both the man and the woman to keep them on check. This is the reason I began by insisting we get knowledge, because it is the principal thing we need here. knowledge is the broker.

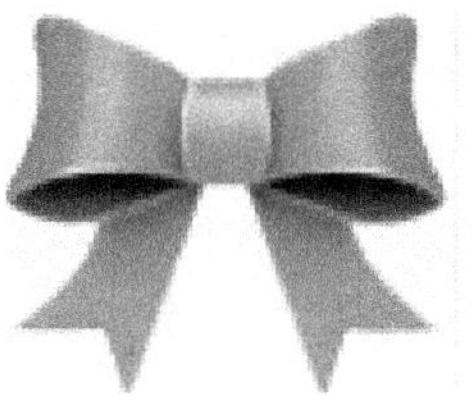

CHAPTER THREE

SIMPLE PROCEDURES

Timing of intercourse is very important during the menstrual circle. Know your wife circle, join her to count the days so you too will be carried along. Ask, what day is she in, so both of you will time your intercourse close to the ovulation day.

The reason is because the XY sperms are faster in movement, they get to the egg first. e.g. if you had sex three days before ovulation, you have the chance of conceiving a girl child. Because the XY sperms tend to die quick, but the XX sperms remain for a longer time and bigger in quantity, whenever the egg is released they can still be fertilized.

However, having sex close to ovulation day is better at least 2 days before or few days after ovulation is better for conceiving a boy.

The woman's body generate acidic environment that allow speed flow of sperm when dropped. So adequate romance is required to make her vagina wet before ejaculation.

Positioning for intercourse, deep penetration is required here because of the PH, it helps place the sperms closer to the egg, this places the sperms close to the egg for fertilization. Shallow penetration which in some cases, leads to ejaculation that the dropping will end up not getting inside. The aggressive sperms that produces boy, because it does not live long, ends up not getting close to the egg, and at the end it favours a girl.

The woman should be helped to reach orgasm before ejaculation, this help her body to release alkaline substances that makes the environment favours a boy.

For a male child, try to space your sex days, at least three to four days to build your sperm count.

The two key aspect to watch out for in this study is the ovulation day and menstrual circle counting,

Watch out for the day and count the circle properly.

Don't forget that children are God's own gift. He gives children, it's not the making of any one. What we are teaching is simply following the rules guiding child bearing as God put them in a woman's system. Don't ever think that you are the one that makes it happen. No, God does!

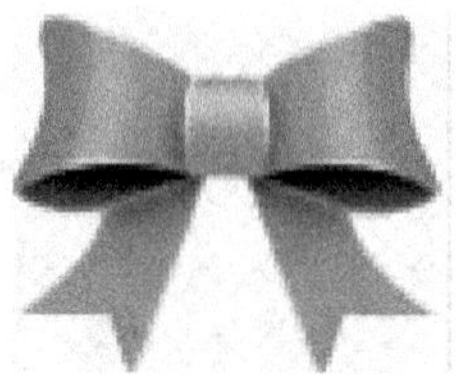

CHAPTER FOUR

DON'T RUSH HER

Don't have sex with her when she is angry.

Avoid sex when she is irritated or sick.

Avoid sex when she is not properly aroused and stimulated.

Avoid sex when she is suffering from painful experience.

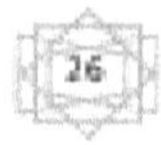

Avoid sex when she is unstable emotionally and not ready for sex.

Avoid sex when she is experiencing a fearful moment.

what to do to help the woman reach orgasm.

Make sure you take her through enough foreplay, touching various part to help her aroused and ready.

Don't just rush in and ejaculate and stand immediately.

In the case of looking for a male child after ejaculation stay in there for some time to allow the sperm to settle in before you stand up from her.

God bless your home; I look forward to hearing your testimonies.

CAN THIS RELATIONSHIP WORK?
WAYS TO FIND OUT

1. In real relationships, you will experience unselfish caring about the interest of one another, interest of another comes first.

While in wrong relationship, it is selfish, restrictive and concentration is on what the

other person is doing for the other as a yardstick to measure the love.

2. In real relationships, romantic feelings start gradually,

But in wrong relationship, it starts immediately and so it will end the moment he/she gets what is being looked for.

3. In real relationship, the attraction is on the total personality and quality of the person even after wedlock.

While in wrong relationship, interest is built on the facial out look of the person, physical appearance, personality and ambitions of the person is not a concern. Attention are on. Does he own a car, house, good job and her bodily outlook? Most likely to experience a delayed marriage.

4. In real relationship, waiting for a real love makes you a better person, chances of making mistake is slim. Because such person will advise and correct you when you are wrong, will support you morally and financially to achieve the goals you have.

Wrong relationship abandons when in distress and difficulty, distractive and disorganizing. Disowns when in challenges, especially financial challenges.

5. Real relationship sees the other person faults, yet still loves him/her. Looks out to what to do to make the other person becomes what he/she expects

Wrong relationship is not real, it sees itself as perfect, ignore negative traits that could make the relationship to crash in future, overlooking nagging doubts and personality flows which the person refuses to stop or change.

These signs are the things to watch out for when looking for real and true love for marriage. Be careful when he rushes you for marriage, courtship must be observed, at least three months before the wedlock.

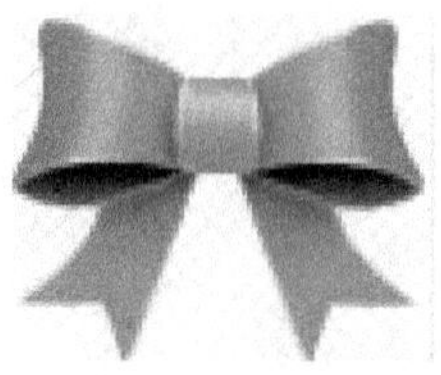

CHAPTER FIVE

WHAT MAKES A SUCCESSFUL MARRIAGE?

" Wives, likewise, be submissive to your own husbands, that even if some do not obey the word, they, without a word, may be won by the conduct of their wives, when they observe your chaste conduct accompanied by fear. Do not let your adornment be merely outward--arranging the hair, wearing gold, or putting on fine apparel, rather let it be the hidden person of the heart, with the incorruptible beauty of a gentle and quiet spirit, which is very precious in the sight of God. For in this manner, in former times, the holy women who trusted in God also adorned themselves, being submissive to their own husbands, as Sarah obeyed Abraham, calling him lord, whose daughters you are if you do good and are not afraid with any terror. Husbands, likewise, dwell with them with understanding, giving honor to the wife, as to the weaker vessel, and as being heirs together of the grace of life, that your prayers may not be hindered." 1 peter 3:1-7 NKJV

The word 'place' as mentioned, is a successful home.
Submission to husband, and understanding of the wife as weaker vessel, are instrumental to building this successful home.

When a woman submit to her husband as her 'lord' (Sarah, as a case study) and the man understand the wife's weaknesses as an imperfect person, both become 'co' in actualization of their objectives in marriage. Paul says, "Wives submit to your own husband as to the Lord", Ephesians. 5:22

Women, who do not submit to the Lordship of Jesus Christ over them, will find it difficult to submit to a husband.

To submit, means to accept, agree, subdue and subject in obedience, it means lowering one's life for the sake of the "head", it means to die to self. Philippians. 2:3-4, Hebrew. 13:17.

Wives should submit to their own husband as to the Lord. This is to say that the woman in question had been submitting to the Lordship of Jesus Christ before now, as Lord and her saviour.

The scripture speaks of the love for the Lord by Timothy grandmother Lois and his mother Eunice, women who submitted to the Lordship of Jesus Christ. "I have been reminded of your sincere faith, which first lived in your grandmother Lois and in your mother Eunice and, I am persuaded, now lives in you also" 2Timothy. 1:5. NIV.

Another person is Ruth. "Then Orpah kissed her mother-in-law good-by, but Ruth clung to her. But Ruth replied, "Don't urge me to leave you or to turn back from you. Where you go I will go, and where you stay I will stay. Your people will be my people and your God my God. Where you die I will die, and there I will be buried. May the Lord deal with me, be it ever so severely, if anything but death separates you and me". Ruth 1:14,16-17

A woman's commitment, character, submissive will lead to all kinds' of open doors for her family, Ruth was a virtuous woman.

Powerful words that **VIRTUOUS** Represents. Check if they are found in you.

V-Very
I-Intelligent woman,
R-Reserved and
T-Trust worthy,
U-Useful.
O-Orderly at home
U-Understanding and
S-Supportive.

It takes a woman who understands the headship of Jesus Christ over the church, to ascribe same to her husband. As it states, "Wives, submit to your husbands as to the Lord. For the husband is the head of the wife as Christ is the head of the church, his body, of which he is the Savior. Now as the church submits to Christ, so also wives should submit to their husbands in everything." Ephesians 5:22-24

Another woman is Anna, a virgin before she got married, she was dedicated to the service of God, committed to religious duties.

Christians are the "church" of Jesus Christ, if we find it difficult to submit to Christ "leadership" in obedience, righteousness, service, good example and proving to the world that we have met with Jesus Christ, others will not come into the church.

THREE REASONS TO SUBMIT TO YOUR HUSBAND

(1) Submission is an obligatory duty of the woman;
it does not mean that the woman is inferior to

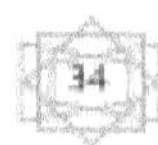

the man. Christian husband and wife are one in Christ. Galatians 3:28.

The word submits, means to subdue and subject   in.
The Christian woman should see it that it is the will of God for her to submit to her husband. 1 peter3:1, 1 Timothy.3:11, Colossians. 3:18. It is not an archaic, outdated and an old fashioned thing as some people think or take it to be.

(2) Submission is an opportunity. vs 1-2. Opportunity to win an unsaved husband to Christ.
God uses it as a powerful spiritual influence in a home. An unsaved husband will not be converted by preaching or nagging in the home. Christian wife who choose to preaching with words to convert their husband and are submissive to them, only drive them farther away from home. 1 Corinthians. 7:16.

3) Submission is ornament. vs 3-6. Peter warns the Christian women not to major on external decoration, but internal character like Abigail in 1Samuel. 25: 14-22. Her husband was an insolent, rude and contentious man,

BUT she was beautiful, intelligent, and intuitive.

We should not choose to imitating the world, worldliness to win our husband. A Christian woman who cultivates the beauty of the inner person, will not have to depend on cheap external things, God is concerned about values and not prices. Character is a hidden part of any human being, which spills out like perfume when it meets with opportunity.

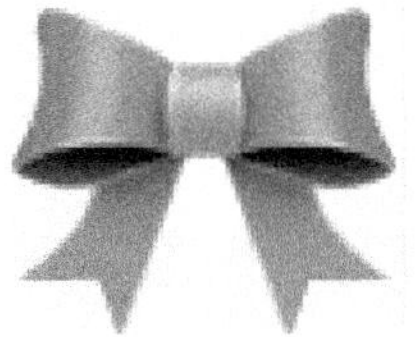

CHAPTER SIX

TRUE RELATIONSHIP, CHRISTIAN PERSPECTIVE
ROMANS 12: 9-21

This requires active involvement in doing what is good, expression of love through a sympathetic care towards one another. These include those who hate you. Evil must be allowed to die, using good deeds as weapons to fight. Paul shows us that, as

Christians we are different in various ways, such as;

Our functions are not the same. Each person is peculiar in his own way, and God his maker loves him/her the way he is. Paul's instructions to Christians came as a result of the need to "love" vs. 9-10; he emphasizes more of these issues in chapter 13: 8-10. He talked about God's attitude towards man and man's attitude towards God and thier neighbours.

He says that God's love for man is not caused by anything we can offer him, we too should love our fellow human being, irrespective of what they are, good or bad, friendly or offensive. Our love for others is to show that we ourselves were loved of God.

10 KEY ISSUES TO AVOID AND TO CLING UPON
1 Avoid hypocrisy, be true and not fake in your endeavours
2 Be loyal to your fellow workers, treat others as brothers and sisters and hate evil'

3 Consider others more desirable than yourselves, respect the desires of others above your own.

4 Be friendly, welcoming, generous, agreeable, look for ways to meet the needs of those around you, as they run to you for help.

5 Return good for the evil done to you, act, don't react, when people hurts you.

6 Share with the feelings of others, in failure or success.
7 Be open minded toward others, allow people to connect with you, don't be selfish.

8 Treat everyone with respect, respect is reciprocal, it is a compliment we all need.

9 We must do it, as long as it concern's peace, work out modalities to see that peace follows you wherever you go.

10 Avoid retaliation (revenge), allow God to judge for us, our duty is to show love.

"Finally, then make my joy complete by being like-minded, having the same love, being one

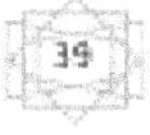

in spirit and purpose. Do nothing out of selfish ambition or vain conceit, but in humility consider others better than yourselves. Each of you should look not only to your own interests, but also to the interests of others. Your attitude should be the same as that of Christ Jesus: Who, being in very nature God, did not consider equality with God something to be grasped, but made himself nothing, taking the very nature of a servant being made in human likeness" Philippians 2:2-7 (NIV)

"Let no one deceive you with empty words, for because of such things God's wrath comes on those who are disobedient. Therefore, do not be partners with them." Ephesians 5:6-7 (NIV).

If Paul could say that his joy will be complete, just because we live in unity, then know that God will be happier to see that we live at peace with one another. Not just live in unity but in a total atmosphere of peace and unity.

We must avoid selfishness, those things which separate us and pursue righteousness and humility, run from hate and rancour, God is against those who instill disunity among his people in disobedience.

Do you know that Jesus is coming back? if you do, what are you doing to see that you are not cut off from those who will be with Him in eternity?

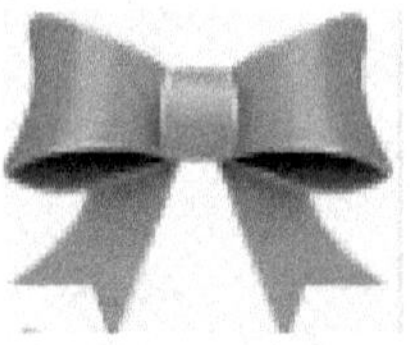

CHAPTER SEVEN

PUT YOUR TRUST
IN GOD

"Whoever believes on Him will not be put to shame." Roman 10:11

God's call to all men is to believe, trust and have faith in Jesus Christ, because if they do not believe it is not his fault.

As Paul was addressing the Gentiles Christians in his letter to the Romans, he was concerned about his own people the Jews, when he saw the grace of God at work in the gentiles.

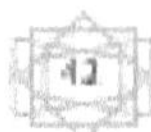

He used it as an emphasis to prove to the gentiles that God's salvation does not depend on man's desire or effort, but on God's mercy. (Romans 9:16).

Paul said that, God's word has not failed, but the Israelites failed, because they did not put their trust in Christ. (Romans.9: 6-7).

Paul described their failure as follows: 1 They tried to reach God by way of law, instead of faith (Romans. 9:30; 10:4).

2 Israel had every opportunity to believe, but has refused to do so, because of disobedience and an obstinate heart (Romans.10:14; 21)

He described to them that the way of faith is easy, and is clearly revealed in Jesus (Romans. 10: 5-13).

Because of this Christ became a stumbling block to them. (Romans 9:33).

Here Paul tries to bring out in clear terms what the prophet Isaiah prophesied many years ago about Jesus Christ. (Isaiah. 28:16), to confirm his message in Romans 9:33.

He described to them that the way of faith is easy and is clearly revealed in Jesus. (Romans. 1o: 4-13)

His emphases were that

1 Those who believe in Christ, however, find out that Christ is "the end of the Law"

2 Christ possesses perfect relationship with God, and thus has fulfilled the law.

3 Christ brings believers into the same relationship with God, and so end the law as a way to approaching God (Romans.3:21)

Paul said, "Anyone" who believes in Him that is to say that the gospel is for every one there is no exception. Whether (Jew or Gentile).

The gospel must be preached to everyone; hence the promise is that "whosoever" puts his trust in Christ shall not be put to shame.

Note: A man's natural birth neither qualifies nor hinders him from receiving the righteousness that comes by faith.

He further says in Romans 10 :12, there is no distinction between Jews and gentiles Romans 10:13. "Everyone who called shall be saved" he said, the Jews held on to it that there is "distinction", and it was entirely in their "favour."

They say that a gentile will have to become a Jew before he will be saved Acts 15:1-31.

Paul maintained that instead of compelling a Greek to become a legalistic Jew, they rather should drop their legalism and become a believing Greek.

He also maintained that there are no two gospels, one for the Jews and another for the gentiles.
His reasons are

1. That both of them are under the same condemnation "guilty of sin"

2. Both of them have the same need "salvation"
3. There is only but one gospel, which promises the same Lord," who is Lord of all", and is abounding in wealth "goodness" towards all who "call upon him." So therefore, I call upon all who are reading this book to embrace God's gift of salvation instead of struggling to establish our own right way of meeting God's righteousness.

We should put our trust in God's Son Jesus and believe him by faith; all will surely be well with us.

Christ died for us all, the same for the Jews and Gentiles. Romans 10:12-13.

Self-righteousness based on law, "one's own right way of meeting God's demand for salvation". Cannot save anyone.

All we need is "trust" in God's own enablement to reach righteousness.

You have been struggling to fulfill God's demand for salvation on your own; Jesus offers it to you free of charge.

You have been rejected because you have not yet received grace to come out of sin.

The bible says, "Anyone who put his trust in Him will not be put to shame", this includes you, all of us.
If we put our trust in him our faces will always look radiant and will not be covered with shame.

He will save us from trouble when we call upon him
Those who put their in him are blessed, they lack nothing, and those who seek him lack no good thing.

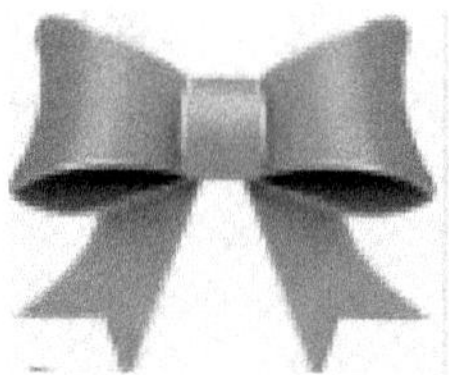

CONCLUSION

Come to Jesus today and forsake your sinful acts along with self-righteousness, and your shame will be over. Scriptures says "if you confess with your mouth, Jesus is Lord, and believe in your heart that God raised him from the dead you will be saved" confess your sin now and put your trust in him.

Your Life is Too Precious

"For God so loved the world, that he gave his only begotten Son, that whosoever believeth in him should not perish, but have everlasting life". John 3:16

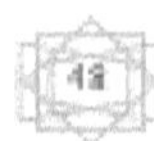

"But God commendeth his love toward us, in that, while we were yet sinners, Christ died for us". Rom 5:8

"And we have seen and do testify that the Father sent the Son to be the Saviour of the world". 1John 4:14

As a sinner you stand to gain nothing by living a sinful life, a life which opposes God's word. Sinful living such as drunkenness, adultery, fornication, lies, wickedness, and such like sinful behaviours, will not take you anywhere. See how God offers you salvation in the name of His Son Jesus Christ as means of escape Romans 5:8

Christ Jesus died while we sinned; but his death was a means to release His blood as atonement for our sins. You are to believe in the blood of Jesus through FAITH in HIM and you will be saved from sin.

Sin is bad and a sinner is the worst enemy of God, again a sinner is subject to condemnation if he/she dies in such state Psalms 29:9-12.

"Gather not my soul with sinners, nor my life with bloody men. In whose hands is mischief, and their right hand is full of bribes. But as for me, I will walk in mine integrity: redeem me, and be merciful unto me. My foot standeth in an even place: in the congregations will I bless the LORD. I testify to you that God initiated a plan to save man and that plan is FAITH in JESUS. Jesus is the ultimate plan of God to save the whole world "And we have seen and do testify that the Father sent the Son to be the Saviour of the world". 1 John 4:14

Why not give your life to Him today and become an ambassador for CHRIST?

About The Author

Rev'd Vincent Uzomah Obibuaku is a preacher of God's Word, Marriage Counselour, Publisher and a Prolific writer, He has authored several books among which are "Singles, Beware Before You Say, I do; Praying in the Spirit; Jesus Came to Set the Captives Free".

He holds B. A (Hons) Christian Theology, Bachelor of Theology (BTh) and Diploma in Theology (DTh) respectively.

<u>OTHER BOOKS BY THE AUTHOR</u>

JESUS CAME TO SET THE CAPTIVES FREE

https://a.co/d/hOnLSM1

"Jesus Came to Set the Captives Free" is a compelling and spiritually uplifting book that explores the profound message of liberation found in the teachings of Jesus Christ. Written by an author deeply rooted in Christian faith, this book delves into the transformative power of Jesus' ministry, emphasizing his mission to free individuals from various forms of captivity, whether they are physical, emotional, or even spiritual.

Drawing on biblical passages, personal experiences, and real-life examples, this book provides readers with a profound understanding of how faith in Jesus can bring about freedom and healing. It offers guidance on overcoming life's challenges, breaking free from bondage, and finding a deeper connection with spirituality. "Jesus Came to Set the Captives Free" is an inspiring read for those seeking spiritual growth and a renewed sense of purpose in their faith journey.

ISBN:

978-978-983-318-4

THE CATCHUMEN

https://a.co/d/6jCTNrU

This is a thoughtfully crafted book that serves as a comprehensive guide to the fundamental principles and teachings of Christianity, through the lens of catechism. Designed to engage both newcomers and those seeking a deeper understanding of Christian faith, it offers a clear and accessible exploration of core beliefs, doctrines, and practices. This follow-up guide takes you on a transformative journey, breaking down complex issues into relatable, digestible segments. It delves into the significance of catechism, revealing its role as a time-honored method for imparting Christian education and nurturing spiritual growth. Whether you are a catechumen, a lifelong believer, or someone simply curious about religious doctrine, this book provides a valuable resource for deepening your understanding of faith. It is an indispensable companion for anyone on a journey to explore, question, and strengthen their spiritual beliefs through the time-tested wisdom of catechism.

THE WEAPON

https://a.co/d/2zktaLv

The efficacy of weapon can be seen in its ability to pull down strongholds and help in gaining a fearless stand against opposing enemies. The battle of life is not fought with bear hands, but with spiritual armour. You cannot imagine the amazing impact prayer through God's weapons of war had against a feeble human and spiritual enemies constantly fighting us, with the intention to destroy our livelihoods. Weapons are used to increase the efficacy and efficiency of activity. Therefore, this book details ways to engage the enemies in battle; though the use of tactical prayers that guarantees victory at the end.

Singles, Beware Before You Say I Do

https://a.co/d/31WRYqR

"Singles, Beware Before You Say I Do" is a practical guidebook designed to provide invaluable advice and wisdom to individuals contemplating marriage.

Written by a seasoned relationship expert, it delves into the essential aspects of choosing a life partner, highlighting potential pitfalls, and providing strategies for making informed decisions before taking the plunge into matrimony.

He used images and diagrams to explain the concept of the conflict between the sinful nature and the Spirit guidance as recorded in the Bible, to give clarity of the traits you expect

to see in an individual before making up your mind in marrying him, in regards to your beliefs and preferences.
Even if you're single and contemplating marriage or simply interested in understanding the complexities of modern relationships.
This book is for you because it provides the knowledge and tools necessary to build strong, lasting, and fulfilling relationships.

The Greedy, Creditor Christian

https://a.co/d/aeU675N

This is a story about quest for wealth and greed, an unscrupulous creditor, driven by avarice was redeemed. Well knowledgeable about God, yet he appears as the quintessential villain, exploiting every opportunity he has to amass riches at the expense of others. His unquenchable thirst for wealth leaves a trail of broken lives and shattered dreams in its wake. But beneath the veneer of unbridled avarice lies the potential for redemption that this gripping story explores. His life later took a dramatic turn when confronted with the consequences of his actions, the wreckage he's left behind. He embarks on an unexpected journey of self-discovery and transformation. You will find yourself captivated by this characters greed, and be grappled with your own conscience. To realize that there's more to life than the relentless pursuit of riches.

www.ingramcontent.com/pod-product-compliance
Lightning Source LLC
Chambersburg PA
CBHW071112260726
48661CB00006B/2592